Home Health 101

Dominic Ottaviano

Self Guide to Home Health Care
and Caregiver Management

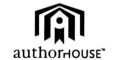

authorHOUSE™

1663 LIBERTY DRIVE, SUITE 200
BLOOMINGTON, INDIANA 47403
(800) 839-8640
WWW.AUTHORHOUSE.COM

First published by AuthorHouse 09/27/05

ISBN: 1-4208-8181-7 (sc)

Printed in the United States of America
Bloomington, Indiana

This book is printed on acid-free paper.

Dedicated
to the memory of:

Florence Krieger
1924-1993

My grandmother who was taken too early by Breast Cancer. Thank you for all the fun I had with you as a child and spending so much time with me. Spend as much time as you can with your grandparents as they are your biggest blessing and the one you will most likely have the least amount of time with so get as much wisdom from them as fast as you can and really appreciate what they have to teach you about yourself. Please remember to support Relay for Life

John Varholick
1943-1995

I was definitely a Dennis the Menace growing up and he was my Mr. Wilson. I can't thank him enough. Folk's be there for your neighbors kids because you really do make a difference. John, may they have a Harley Davidson in heaven and let you lead the ride.

Tom and Minnie Ottaviano
1912 & 1917 - 2000

My Great Aunt and Uncle with which I was blessed to have in my life, truly the perfect example that love can last a lifetime, you will be missed.

Acknowledgements:

Author- Dominic Ottaviano
Editor- Mike Valentino
Cover Design- Jason Dennard
Introduction- Zen Garcia

Special Thanks:

Dominic II and Marisa - My kids, you are the two most important people in my life and give me the inspiration to do everything that I do. You both amaze me in everything you do and know that you are both very awesome people who I love very much.

Monique- The mother of my children, I can not thank you enough for raising Dominic and Marisa to be the wonderful people they are becoming. You have worked very hard to ensure they have a great childhood and I thank you for that. You have done a wonderful job as a mother and that is evident in everything they do and every compliment they receive.

Mom- Thank you for being a wonderful mother and raising me to be the dreamer I am. I know that it drives you crazy and scares you but all my adventures are just that, adventures and I am having fun doing them.

Dad- Sorry for all the headaches but I had fun giving them to you. Thank you for a great childhood and being there for me. More than anything thank you for joining Indian Guides; I really think that made a big difference in guiding my life.

Grandpa Krieger and Grandma and Grandpa Ottaviano- Thank you all for bring our family into the world and giving it the guidance to succeed. I know I am not around as much as I wish but know you are all in my thoughts and prayers all the time.

Anthony and Alyssa- My brother and sister, I love you both very much and wish I would have been around more when you were growing up and more of a big brother. I hope I can be there more in the future if you ever need me; you are both very impressive people.

Brad and Sara- My brother "in-law" and sister "in-law," all I can say is forget the "in-law" part you are now family and thank you for completing Tony and Alyssa. All four of you make awesome aunts and uncles to my children, Thank you.

Ron Starcher- My longest friend, since we were five, I hope we continue to come up with things to get in trouble like when we were younger.

Eric King- All I can say is we have very few true friends in life and I am proud to have you as one of mine, here's to all the good times.

Beth Hartman- We have shared many great times and I thank you for all the listening you have done over the years.

Zen Garcia- Thank you for introducing me to the disability world and allowing me an outlet for helping others.

Carolyn Lacy- Thanks for believing in the new guy and giving me the chance you did back in the beginning. Here's too many more years of having fun and getting stuff done at the same time, what a great little lesson I have learned from you.

Jimmy Selph- Thank you for all you have done in being my mentor; whether you knew it or not you are my mentor and I appreciate all the guidance you have giving me even though I do not always listen, ask my parents, they can also relate to that.

Jason Dennard- Thank you for applying your talents to the cover of this book and for being a great friend

Rick Rose- Thank you for teaching me to fly, may every student find a flight instructor with your patients and perspective to help them accomplish such a challenging goal as you did for me.

Jeff and Debi Shetterly- To my long distance friends, thanks for all the motivation and here's to hoping this really is a small world and getting to see you guys often.

Richard Anthony- Truly a great friend, thanks for all the support over the years.

Mike Valentino- Thank you for all your help and guidance in making this project a success.

Preface
I am home - now what?

It is an overwhelming and mentally draining task for those who deal with home bound issues and this book is written to alleviate the issues and hopefully offer solutions to the common problems and create new possibilities that the freedom of living at home may offer. Whether you are the person living independently or are struggling with having a loved one facing the possibility of institutional living the following pages should help you make the right decision if home living is right for you and then help you succeed with your decision.

You must start by being totally honest and realize independent living can be one of the biggest struggles in life as well as it can be just as rewarding. We must be realistic with the limitations of our self and our surroundings. Doug a client of mine who I met in a nursing home is a great example of the limitations we must accept.

I met Doug at a nursing home with Mark Johnson, an independent living coordinator, as Doug was interviewing me to coordinate his caregiver staff. Doug within a year of my age, around thirty at the time, and a really cool guy. He was a quadriplegic and had very little movement in his arms. At least every hour Doug would need to be coughed, as he had no control of his abdominal muscles so the most taken for granted task of just choking was impossible. A caregiver would have to push on his abdomen while he exhaled to force the air from his lungs and cause the coughing action.

Doug was only allocated twelve hours of home care by the state, which would be impossible for Doug, as he needed more extent care. Mark came up with a plan in which we would find a caregiver to cover the extra hours by staying with Doug at night in trade for free rent. This is a great tactic in most situations but with Doug the night care was to extent and did not allow the evening person any sleep so they could not keep the pace of a second job needed to support themselves. We started having issues with the caregivers not getting enough sleep and could not get back-up care as there were no funds for these extra hours.

The biggest issue for Doug was the lack of support from his family, they were not willing to help and thought that the care provider company should be responsible for ensuring the plan worked. This would be a great theory in a perfect world but as great as this world is it is not perfect. The extra hours are Doug's final responsibility and should include the support of his family. They were unwilling to provide any emergency care for Doug and only added to the problems by creating issues with the caregiver staff.

These problems progressed until Doug was unable to continue independent living and was forced back to the nursing home. Two months after returning to the nursing home Doug passed, as do most people forced into institutional living. Could Doug have succeeded at independent living? With a supportive family or state funding to provide the extra hours of care needed by Doug I feel he could have been much more successful and probably been much happier.

We must carefully weigh our strengths and limitations and the limitations of our environment including our friends and family. Be honest with yourself and find strength in the ideas of this book and knowing thousands of individuals are facing and succeeding at the issues facing you today.

CONTENTS

Preface
I am home - now what?   xiii

Introduction
By Zen Garcia   1

Chapter One
Home care vs. the nursing home   7

Chapter Two
Hiring Caregivers   19

Chapter Three
Pay, Benefits, and Workers Compensation   29

Chapter Four
Staffing and Interviewing your Caregivers   37

Chapter Five
Problem Solving andEffective Communication   47

Chapter Six
Daily routine and scheduling   57

Chapter Seven
Plan of Care and Putting It To Use   65

Chapter Eight
Activities to get involved with   75

Chapter Nine
Family Assistance   83

Chapter 10
Home Monitoring and Safety   91

Introduction
By Zen Garcia

My friend Dominic Ottaviano and I have been great friends for a long time now. Though he personally does not have a disability, I know that he understands disability with more depth than most. Through our friendship he has seen first-hand how much quadriplegia impacts a person's life. I have been a quadriplegic for 10 years now, having incurred my disability when a van I got a ride in lost its brakes on a California mountain road; we plunged 85 feet to the ground. Lucky to have survived, I have spent the last decade learning about disability culture, where we are, and how far we still have to go. In truth, people with disabilities are still in the process of defining what it means to be disabled now, in modern times, with the help of the Americans with Disabilities Act, and new accessibility. With more and more young people surviving traumatic experiences, we are no longer just a culture content with being placed in the closets and living in the shadows of society. There is fire to justify more change.

I had been an advocate for three years when I met Dominic through my girlfriend Traci. He was then running a limo service, driving for hire while getting his pilot's license and finishing his degree. He had a ten-year history in several business and insurance ventures. For weeks Dom came by to hang out and talk; soon long-term care became the focus of our conversations. I found myself rambling on and on about the lack of good providers, the bias in the governor's budget, the Unlock the Waiting List campaign, and how it all tied together with a history of genocide and institutional care.

I spoke of my affiliation with ADAPT and what they were doing to change the current system. I told him how I wanted to open up my own company and do things for my friends and self, but couldn't because of regulations. I wanted to create something that would benefit all involved leaving no one out and be a win-win for everybody. I thought he listened because he just wanted to be my friend and did not truly hear what I was saying.

But then a month later Dominic met and got hired by Jimmy Selph, doing insurance and payroll for a company called Southeastern Administrative Services. SAS turned out to be the missing link in the puzzle of providing good long-term care in Georgia. A couple weeks later I found myself having lunch with Jimmy, his daughter Tracy Simpson, her husband Sandy Simpson, and Dominic to talk a little more in detail about the things I've been ranting and raving about for years.

Dominic and I recognized that there was a way to cater to the long term care system, which maintained people's identities and dignity and served them in their own homes while at the same time upholding profitability for a company. So I spoke about the 1999 United States Supreme Court decision Olmstead vs. LC/EW which upheld Title II of the Americans with Disabilities Act maintaining a person's right to live life in "the most integrated setting" of society and how because of this decision states were being forced to set up comprehensive plans to move people out of nursing homes and into the community as well as move Medicaid dollars away from nursing homes and into community home based services. I guess I was convincing because it was soon after that that we conversed about pooling our resources together to do and create something that would benefit the disability community.

Explaining the numbers, they were sold on the idea of doing something that not only would allow them to make money, but would also allow them to do a tremendous amount of good where a tremendous amount of good was needed. Knowing long-term care would be an area of business that would not disappear anytime soon, they thought it would be a good area to place investment.

As a recipient of the waiver I had seen the long term care program in Georgia through many changes and found that I had more difficulty dealing with bad providers than I did dealing with my disability. I knew things could be a lot better and that the only reason they had stayed like this for so long is because we had still been in the process of developing the structure for care. Because there was minimal if any competition at the time, bad providers were able to assume a monopoly and dictate how they think home care should be. There were no alternatives at the time in many regions to the provider who understood they could do whatever they wanted because there was no one else to say different. And so, in 2000, after a year delay accessing necessary permits, they were able to open Calle Vinas, Inc., a home care provider. It was then that Dominic spent the next year going out and meeting with clients and case managers setting up the framework that is Calle Vinas today.

In 2 years Calle Vinas became the largest provider in Georgia providing care that upheld the Independent Living Philosophy. We knew future long term care must seek to educate and inspire individuals to dream, to seek out goals which allow them to get ahead, possibly propelling self into the job market so that in becoming part of the system, they/we start giving back to programs which may assist others to a renewed sense of identity and dignity. Long Term Care should not be maintenance but growth, evolution, change, inclusion. It should shoot to serve disabled individuals with quality service to create a healthy environment ripe to inspire. With the focus of the Independent Living Philosophy in mind and consumer directed care, Long Term Care becomes empowerment to hope. People with disabilities need that in life to reclaim parts of self lost in accidents incurring disability. In nursing homes people become patients and patients become burdens to employees who cannot cater to the needs and whims of the many assigned to their care.

With community based services people with disabilities are able to interact with creation and humanity, and in that way learn the lessons that life has to relate to us all, those lessons which will cause us to evolve as human beings, and help our souls to whatever purpose serves fulfillment. Doesn't everybody deserve that? Don't we all have that right, simply because we were born, to experience life in whatever way we choose, no matter how that may be, whether or not others accept our life and way of living as "worthy?" Life is beautiful in its blessings, a miracle in its unfolding, glorious in its touch; and all persons, all children, all individuals should be allowed to kiss it softly, sweetly, and drink from its lips, all wisdom, all knowledge, and all experience.

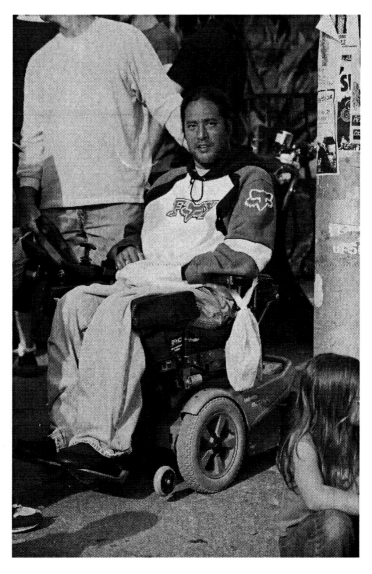

Zen Garcia at the Little Five Points Halloween Parade

<u>NOTES</u>

Chapter One
Home care vs. the nursing home

Let me begin by saying there are some really good, honest, hard working people out there taking care of the elderly and the infirm in nursing homes. They perform thankless jobs on a daily basis, and many of them are true angels of mercy. I don't want to demean these people or their profession in any way. It is not always the caregivers who are bad; they are understaffed. However, if you are faced with the choice of homecare vs. going into a nursing home, in my opinion it's a no-brainer: stay home!

There are a number of reasons why I feel so strongly about this. First and foremost, I have been to a number of nursing homes and I have seen for myself what goes on there. In many of them, the patients are basically "warehoused." By that I mean there is little or no personal attention given to their psychological and emotional needs. It's as if society has forgotten that these are *human beings*. No matter how old you are, no matter how sick you are, you never stop being human. You should receive all of the respect and dignity that other people (i.e., the young and healthy) not only have come to expect, but demand.

But once you step inside a nursing home, it's like it's a different world. I hate to say it because it's such a grim analogy, but in many ways it's like entering inside the gates of a prison. There's a feeling of confinement, of being cut off from the outside world. And it's such a sad place. Just walk inside and you will immediately notice that there are many people sitting around in wheelchairs, just waiting to die. It's mostly old people, but there are some younger ones too, usually severely disabled. The smell is not very pleasant to say the least. The one thought most people (of any age) have after spending even a little time in a nursing home is, *Man, please don't let me ever end up in one of these places*!

There is a bill wending its way through Congress right now that will make states match what they pay for nursing homes to what they pay for home care programs. You should do all you can to see that it passes. It is called the Community Attendant Services and Supports Act (MiCASSA), Senate Bill 1935, authored by ADAPT (American Disabled for Attendant Programs Today). It allows Medicaid funds to be shifted from nursing homes to Home and Community-Based programs.

OK, so we can see that the nursing home is clearly a place you want to avoid. That's easy…if you're rich! But what about the rest of us? How does the average man or woman who becomes incapacitated (either by illness or by advanced age) afford <u>not</u> to go into the nursing home? I have some good news for you: home care is not some sort of impossible dream. There are indeed ways to receive the proper medical care and assistance that you need right in your own home. Many different factors will determine whether or not this is a viable option. Let's take a closer look.

The first question you need to answer is, how many hours of assistance will you (or your ailing loved one) need to successfully be cared for at home. Don't just throw out the first arbitrary number that pops into your head. Think this out carefully. Be realistic about the person's needs. One scenario might be dealing with an elderly person. For the sake of argument, let's say it's your grandmother. Precisely what kind of assistance does she require? Maybe she has trouble seeing and you simply need someone to help her with the cooking, and with bathing so she doesn't hurt herself. In this case, you can figure out approximately how many hours a week you will need a home care visit to help with these specific tasks.

That's one end of the spectrum. The easier part. On the other end, there will be people who will require a much greater amount of assistance. People with severe disabilities such as quadriplegia would certainly fit into this category. These are people who have suffered from some sort of spinal cord injury. They may have various levels of paralysis. Some, for example, can move their arms, but not their hands or wrists. But the common problem for all of these people is that they need help with almost all facets of daily living. This includes lots of basics that most of us take for granted, such as taking a shower or even feeding yourself. Severely disabled people face a variety of problems you probably never even thought of. For example, when they sleep they need to be turned; otherwise they will develop bed sores and other problems. Of course, they have virtually no control over their bodily functions, so they wear a bag (connected to a catheter) to collect the urine their bodies produce, and it has to be drained every morning. Naturally, they can't do this themselves. Furthermore, when it's time to get out of bed, somebody has to lift this person into the wheelchair, roll him into the shower, etc.

I won't be overly graphic, but you need to also realize that severely disabled people often need somebody to help them eliminate solid bodily wastes too. This is done usually every other day.

The variety of tasks facing a severely disabled person's caregiver is almost endless. Getting the person dressed, brushing his teeth and a million other things. All sorts of everyday things. In females, there would also be feminine bodily issues to deal with. Of course, if you or your loved one is female, you should always have a female caregiver. Yes, it's illegal to hire somebody based on gender. But this is not a major problem since the vast majority of caregivers (probably 95%) are female. In any case, the last thing you want is for an unattended disabled female to be left alone with a male caregiver. That leaves her in a vulnerable situation and opens up a number of sexual issues that should be avoided at all costs.

When trying to determine how many hours of care you or your loved one will require each week, don't make the mistake of underestimating how long each individual task can take. For example, getting dressed. If you're an able bodied person, you can probably get yourself dressed in five minutes or less. But trying to dress somebody else is an altogether different proposition. It can take a very long time. Take into account how difficult it is to remove clothing, then have to pull the new clothing onto the other person's body while they can't offer any help. It is a good idea to wear clothes that are slightly loose fitting and made of a more durable material to better handle assisted dressing.

Eating is another everyday task that is so much more difficult with a severely disabled person. Often it means handling the fork and spoon for the disabled person. Mealtimes are, therefore, much longer than they would be for people without this disability. And sometimes eating means using a stomach bag with a tube, which presents its own difficulties. You need to do a little experimenting with all of these everyday living activities and then write down a realistic amount of time for each of them.

Now, you also need to realize that there are many tasks that aren't directly related to physical needs. For example, house cleaning. For someone taking care of certain elderly people, it may just be a few things that need to be attended to (dirty laundry, dishes, etc.). On the opposite extreme, again, let's say for someone who is completely dependent, it will be necessary for a caretaker to do *everything* around the house. Obviously, a person with a severe disability won't be capable of barely any of the ordinary tasks that we all do around the house every day. We will go into this in more detail in the chapter on daily routine and scheduling.

Clearly, for these people the only kind of home care that will be adequate will have to be 24 hour care. And keep in mind that in all likelihood the caregiver will also have to do things like cutting the grass and other minor (but time-consuming) maintenance around the house. Of course, a job such as this could also be done by a landscaper, or (better for the budget) by a family member. My point is, don't overlook any of these "minor" things; they can become a big problem if you and your family don't do some thinking and planning ahead of time.

In home care situations that require 24 hour assistance, there are usually 3 caregivers who work in shifts. Whoa, you're thinking, that will break the bank! Not necessarily. Let's take a closer look at the numbers, and the kinds of financial assistance that may be available to you. Sometimes we hire people for a flat rate, say $250 for an entire weekend. When you hire someone, you have to pay them salary, plus matching taxes, and worker's comp. I suggest you hire a payroll company and save yourself a lot of headaches. Multiply whatever the caretaker makes (say, $8 per hour) by 50% (for the taxes and worker's comp) and that number increases to $12 per hour. The overall cost, therefore, can be $70,000 a year for someone who needs 24/7 care 365 days a year. We'll have more to say about this in the chapter on staffing and pay.

Now, I'm certain there are many of you who simply could not afford such an amount, even if other family members chipped in. In some cases, however, there may be funds available to help cover these hours. If you are over 65, you won't be eligible for a Medicare program in your state and will be considered a "private pay," meaning you must pay for the caregivers out of your own pocket. Or from insurance, if you were fortunate enough to have bought a policy that covers such expenses. Not all of them do. Be sure to carefully read over all of the terms and conditions of your policy.

If you are over 65, you are covered under the federal program (Medicaid), which is both good and bad. It's good because the government will pay your expenses. But it's bad because Medicaid has *no home health care funding*. So you either have to pay for it yourself or go into the nursing home. Not an enviable situation.

Are there any other solutions? In some cases there might be. For example, for persons under age sixty five there may be independent living funds available from the state. There may also be programs to support home health. These will vary greatly from one state to another. Moreover, although there are not funds available (at least not yet) for persons over age sixty five, there are bills right now in Congress that will hopefully change that.

You may be wondering just how do these programs vary from state to state. It usually depends on what kind of care the disabled person needs. The state might, for example, give money for 8 hours a day. The exact amount will depend on the state's budget and how much its Legislature and Governor allocates for such programs.

Here's the bottom line to the whole issue of keeping down the amount of hours you need to pay for a caregiver (which obviously lowers the amount of money you will need available to afford home care): how much assistance will there be from other family members AND how much can the disabled person reasonably be expected to do for him or herself? For example, will the disabled or elderly person be managing the household himself, or will it be necessary for a family member (brother, sister, son, daughter, etc.) to take on that job? If this individual can maintain a certain level of independence, only use your "emergency" people when you really need them, otherwise you will burn out the people in your support circle (in other words, don't "cry wolf"). I will go into much more detail later in the book when we discuss problem solving.

I suggest that you ask (and answer) these very common yet quite important questions:

Do I have the additional support I will need to run errands?

This would include a number of things (groceries, fixing the car, taking the dog to the vet, etc.) that the disabled or elderly person might not be able to do himself. But somebody will still have to do it. If you can designate somebody other than the caregiver, that will cut down the overall hours she will have to be on the payroll.

Do I have someone for emergency backup when there is no caregiver available?

Don't overlook this one. Remember, caregivers have lives and families too. They need breaks (personal time). Vacations. And they get sick. Prepare for all of these contingencies well in advance and don't ever let yourself be caught off guard by unforeseen circumstances.

Is this "back up" person realistic about being called at anytime when a caregiver is not available?

People love to volunteer. Especially when it comes to helping someone with an illness or an injury. It makes them feel good about themselves, and indeed, they should be commended for it. However, some people are more talk than they are action. If at all possible, try to enlist the help of someone who is genuinely reliable and trustworthy. And will be there when needed most.

Am I capable of handling things for myself so I don't put too much pressure on my friends and family for handling these back up hours?

The answer to this one calls for some deep introspection and a lot of honesty. You may *want* to answer "yes," but think about this question in very practical terms. The good intentions of most disabled and elderly people make them not want to "be a burden" on those around them. However, nobody asks to get sick or injured. It just happens. Nobody should ever feel guilty about seeking out adequate care and support.

Am I willing to support my parents at anytime if they are the ones receiving the home health care?

Lots of kids feel a responsibility to do this. But (if you are that kid) again, I urge you, just like your parent, to be realistic about all of this. Remember, you have a life too (spouse, kids, job, home, etc.) and taking care of an elderly parent may mean a lot more work than you ever expected. I'm sure your heart is in the right place. Just make sure your head is too.

Finally, let me conclude this chapter by summarizing the primary benefits of home care vs. going into a nursing home. Most importantly, there is the freedom that comes from independent living. Even if you have a 24 hour caregiver, it still is a boost to your spirit to feel that at least you were able to remain in your own home. That gives people a sense of freedom and dignity they would never have in a nursing home.

Being at home also means that the disabled or elderly person will not have to face the abuse that, unfortunately, has become so rampant in some nursing homes. Many cases have now been well documented where untrained (and certainly uncaring) staff members have physically abused elderly and disabled people. And then there is emotional and verbal abuse, which sometimes can be almost just as nasty and painful. With properly screened, well-trained home caregivers, that kind of intolerable behavior will be one less thing to worry about.

There are other benefits to staying home that you may not have even thought about. For example, persons at home with a disability have a greater connection to the community, which can really help them out psychologically. Also, sometimes the individual facing the nursing home is not old, but is a young person with a disability. And a nursing home is such an awful place for a young person to have to live. It's bad enough for the old.

Finally, put yourself in the shoes of person who is facing this decision. Think about what that nursing home is like. Is that the sort of place where you would want to spend the last years of your life? Wouldn't it be much more comforting to be in the familiar surroundings of your own home? I think the answer to this last question speaks volumes. Let it speak to you.

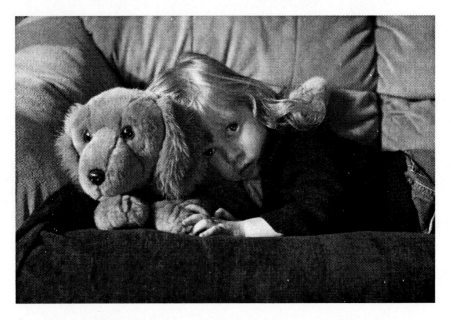

Nora Kieffer at 2 ½; having care at home can be
needed at any age, our thought are with you Nora.

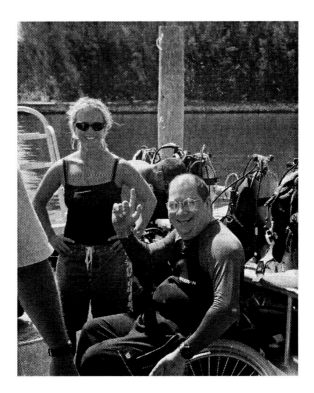

Tony Boatright and Tanja Link Scuba Diving in the Bahamas

NOTES:

Chapter Two
Hiring Caregivers

You have two basic choices when hiring caregivers, you can hire them yourself or go through an agency. Let me give you some solid, based on experience advice. Doing it yourself is not a good option: you have to do all of the work, including proving worker's compensation, making sure they have CPR and First Aid training (and that it is current), doing a background check, and getting a Tax ID number and making quarterly payments to the government. You also have to make matching Social Security payments. Moreover, you have to pay unemployment insurance, both state and federal. Do these sound like the kinds of duties and responsibilities you want to burden yourself with? Probably not. It involves a huge amount of responsibility. There are literally hundreds of details that you would need to be familiar with and accurately keep track of. Not to mention, if the worker makes any mistakes, or messes up in any way (and believe me, there are <u>plenty</u> of ways!) look no further than the mirror to guess who will end up being liable for everything.

My suggestion would be to seek out an agency of some sort. These people are professionals. They are in the business every day and they have a thorough understanding of the rules, regulations and procedures. Hiring caregivers, in my opinion, is not the sort of thing you can "learn as you go." There's very little room for error. Sure, you could attempt to do it on your own, but beware of the risks. For example, I have a friend whose elderly aunt required in home care. Thinking this would be a relatively simple task, he didn't use an agency. He went ahead and hired the first few applicants who answered his newspaper ad. Over the course of the next few months, however, his aunt started noticing that she couldn't find certain things around the house. Her favorite pair of earrings, that her mother had given her on her deathbed, had disappeared. And the $25 gift certificate she had bought for her grandson's birthday was missing too.

Well, my friend assumed that his poor old aunt may have been experiencing the early signs of Alzheimer's Disease. He even brought her to a doctor to check out his hunch, but all the tests came back negative. Then, one day my friend showed up unexpectedly at his aunt's house on his way to work (he needed to use the bathroom). He had a key so he let himself in through the front door. His aunt was asleep on the couch in front of the TV. He smiled as he passed her. But then he heard something as he headed toward the bathroom. He stopped at the doorway to his aunt's bedroom and peered inside. He was stunned to see one of the caregivers rifling through his aunt's jewelry box! He fired her on the spot.

Unfortunately, that's not where the story ended. He had no solid proof. The girl made a lame excuse about dusting the jewelry box. He was sure she was lying, but he had nothing that he could go to the police with. He was just glad to be rid of her. However, the little thief then had the audacity to apply for unemployment. In the end, she got the unemployment and now this unfortunate man has to pay this crook his hard earned money…even though his aunt later passed away. That's right, the way the law is constructed, even though his aunt was deceased, her nephew was still required to continue paying for this dishonest caregiver's unemployment. It's not fair. But that's the way it is.

Here's another reason to use an agency. If you are on a state in home care plan you will most likely be required to choose a support agency to manage your account and pay your people. Moreover, should you qualify for one of the state's "waivers" they will re-route your Medicaid money to in home care. This means you will have to use a state licensed home care provider. Assuming you get on the state's program, they will give you a list of these agencies to choose from.

For a private pay person, someone not on a government program, I recommend using a staffing agency or an employee leasing company. They will be able to help you find people and will also keep you in compliance with state and federal laws as well as tax and unemployment issues.

OK, assuming you are now convinced and you do indeed want to go the agency route, first you need to realize that there are different kinds of agencies. One kind of agency is a temp agency. Some of these specialize in providing medical workers, but not all of them. Some of them may simply be general help temporary agencies. In any case, at the very least you will most likely want to hire a Certified Nursing Assistant (CNA) through the temp agency that you are working with. A temp agency will usually charge a 50% mark-up per employee that they provide you.

One of the biggest drawbacks of using a temporary agency is that you need to do a good deal of the work yourself. These agencies are not licensed by the state, so you're pretty much on your own when it comes to dealing with them. Keep in mind that they will only provide what you ask them for. So don't be timid when it comes to asking specific questions about what you need. This might include a caregiver certified in CPR or First Aid. You also may want to require the worker to take a drug test before your final hiring decision (make sure this is legal in your state, as the laws on this practice vary). Another good idea (and this goes for all three kinds of agencies) is to ask for – and check out – their references.

You will also have to do the interviewing and background checking. And be sure to ask for a Worker's Comp certificate. The rate will be a 50% mark –up on whatever you choose to pay. This will depend in large part on where you are located, as some geographic regions are much more expensive than others. Call a nursing home and ask what they pay their CNAs; as a general rule of thumb, if the local nursing home pays $6.50, you can expect to pay $7.00 or $7.50.

Your best option, and in my opinion the easiest, is to hire the help you need through a home health agency. These agencies are required to be licensed by the state. Accordingly, the caregivers that they send to work for you will have to be certified by the state, so you can rest easier and have confidence in their qualifications. They will be either a CNA or a PCA (Personal Care Assistant). The agency will also do background checks on these individuals as well as make certain that they have been properly trained in CPR and First Aid. Moreover, the agency will also provide back-up, which is important in case a worker isn't able to come in on any given day due to illness or a personal emergency. You can negotiate with the agency, regarding what kind of specific services you will require and for how many hours per week. The pay is also negotiable, to a certain degree. And be sure to ask for a Worker's Comp certificate (see same article as earlier).

There are other important reasons for hiring through a homecare agency. One is that they are likely to have not only the best qualified, but also the most satisfied workers. Why? Because they offer benefits (vacation, health insurance, etc.). This makes for happier employees, who will do a better job.

The third kind of agency you might want to consider is an employee leasing / staffing company. Although some of these are large national companies, you may not be familiar with how they work. In a nutshell, you hire them and they do all of the checking and background work. They do all of the payroll work, almost like a payroll company, but the employee is their employee, which is the big difference. They will negotiate the price with you. They will handle the workers comp rate for homecare workers, which is 10 to 20% of what they pay the worker. And FICA, which, depending on the state you live in, is 10 to 15%. The total is 20 to 35%.

You will also discover that in home care is waived from overtime pay laws. That means there is no legal obligation to pay employees time and a half. The only other job that is waived from overtime, interestingly enough, is offshore fishing.

Of course, there are some serious drawbacks to this option. Most significantly, you have to do your own advertising and interviewing. My recommended philosophy is to hire a *good* person rather than a *trained* person. Why do I say this? Think about it, you can always train a person to do the job but you can't train someone to be a good person. These people will be working very closely with either you or a loved one, and they need to be an individual whom you can trust.

The person you end up hiring may well right now be living just down the street. College students, for example, usually make great caregivers. The main portion of the job only takes about one or two hours, then the rest of the time they are on standby, depending on the coverage you have, which allows the student plenty of study time. They also work well because they tend to be more outgoing, responsible people, which is why they've chosen to advance themselves by attending college. Depending on your age and needs, a college person can make a great caregiver and a fun person to just be around.

Don't be too flustered by the concept of doing your own advertising. It's really not as difficult as you might think. My advice? Put up ads at colleges and clubs frequented by kids from the local universities. Newspapers (including college newspapers) and churches are also ideal places to find caregivers. Of course, these jobs for untrained workers are only applicable for situations where there is no need for anything technical such as working with intravenous or other complex medical equipment. A great web site to post a free ad is www.craigslist.com and click on your community however do not reply on the internet solely; a majority of caregivers do not have access but college students do.

Here is a model for a possible newspaper ad

> Enthusiastic individual needed to assist disabled
> ___1___ in ___2___ area. C.N.A.s and students
> encouraged to apply. ____3___. __4__per
> hour, paid vacation, and paid health insurance.
> Call ___5___ for info.

1. Insert client description i.e.… male, female, student, poet, artist, professional.

2. Insert job location.

3. Insert job hours.

4. Insert hourly pay.

5. Insert phone number.

Please realize, however, that these ads are not one size fits all. In other words, be sure to customize them. One ad might make it clear that the job would involve caring for an elderly man who likes to be read to. Another ad might go in a completely different direction. For example, it might read, "Young, disabled artist needs assistance." By all means, don't just say "disabled person." After all, this person is an individual, and so is the caregiver you are seeking. Wisely use tightly written descriptions to find the best possible match between the caregiver and the person who is seeking assistance.

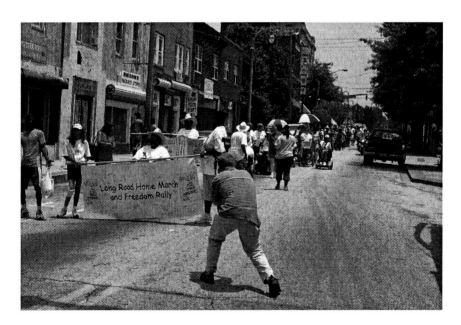

Disability awareness parade in Atlanta

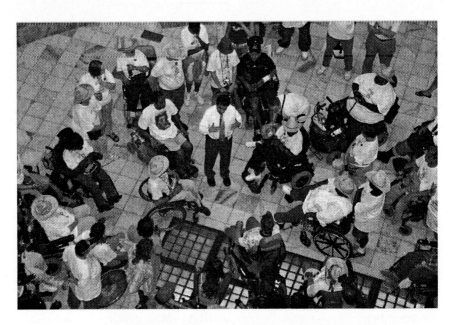

A little more talk with the politicians

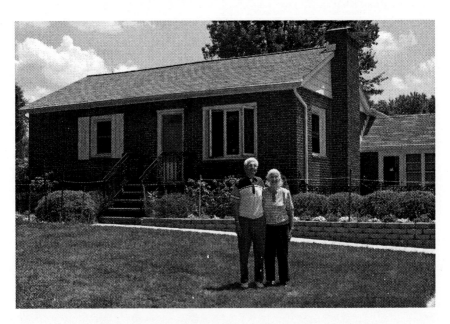

Grandpa and Grandma Ottaviano in the house
they built together, where people should be

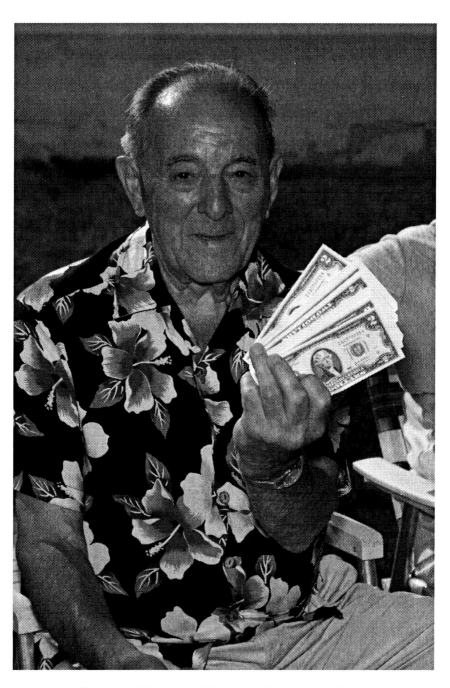

Grandpa Krieger celebrating his 80th birthday

NOTES:

Chapter Three
Pay, Benefits, and Workers Compensation

It's Monday morning. Your caregiver, Jane, shows up bright and early, as always, to assist in getting you ready for the day. You roll in for a hot shower and are thinking of what a great day it's going to be. Suddenly, you hear a loud crash. Horrified, you look over and see that Jane has slipped on some water and lay sprawled on the floor. She moans that her back is really hurting, gets up and limps toward the phone to call 911.

As we all know, accidents can happen at any time. And if you're going to have employees working in your home, you better become well versed in liability issues and how they function. Without Workers Compensation Insurance you could be leaving yourself wide open to a number of costs that might be far heftier than you ever imagined. These could include medical bills, lost wages, and disability compensation if the injury is serious. How do you avoid this unenviable situation? For starters, you need to know whether or not your care provider company is treating your caregivers as subcontractors or as employees. I can't overstate how important this distinction is. You can find out by simply calling and asking them. Also, and just as importantly, you want to find out if your provider carries Workers Comp Insurance for the employees they are sending to your home. If so, request a Certificate of Insurance.

Many Home Health Agencies classify employees as subcontractors to reduce taxes and not pay Workers Comp Insurance. This is a great situation for the agencies as it cuts employee cost by as much as 25%. When dealing with several employees and thousands of hours annually, this translates into a great deal of profit for the agency. Unfortunately, it is a situation of the rich getting richer and the employee getting bitten by the ignorance bug.

By being classified as a subcontractor these workers are responsible for their own "matching taxes" FUTA, SUTA, and FICA. Talk about getting double dipped! Withholding taxes are not taken from the employee's check, which leaves them a huge tax bill at the end of the year while the rest of us are enjoying our refunds. And, although some companies withhold tax in an escrow account, the tax situation for these workers is still far from ideal. As we've seen, the subcontracted caregiver pays more in taxes right off the bat by having to pay the "matching taxes" themselves rather than the employer paying them.

Matching taxes are the Social Security and Unemployment Insurance an employer must pay on all employees. The amount for these taxes in Georgia is 11.15%. I am going to continue to use Georgia's tax numbers as my example. Of course, your state may be different, but this example will give you the information you need for a basic understanding. By classifying caregivers as subcontractors the employer does not have to pay the 11.15% and retains that money as profit. Someone always has to pay when someone else saves, and here is where the caregiver takes the hit.

The caregiver as a subcontractor also has no Unemployment Insurance so if terminated they cannot collect unemployment. With the high turnover rate in this career, the risk of job loss is above average.... and it is the caregiver who takes all the risk. To add insult to injury, the employer is not paying the Social Security employer portion, which the caregiver now has to pay on his or her own nickel at the end of the year. The Social Security rate is 7.65% in addition to all the other taxes that cut into the caregiver's check. There's barely enough left over to get by.

But wait -- it gets worse! We haven't even talked about Workers Comp yet. By classifying the employee as a subcontractor, Workers Compensation insurance is not required by law. The cost savings and increased profits to the agency is staggering; this is pure profit and is an incredible cost cutter. The employee is the one who suffers. And *you*.

Here's the situation: your caregiver has no Unemployment Insurance, and increased taxes through Social Security, while your personal support agency fattens its wallet. No wonder it's so rare to find agencies that do the right thing. Keep in mind that agencies paying the Social Security and Unemployment Taxes have expenses that are not immediately seen by the consumer. You the consumer will not see the 11.15% matching taxes or the 10%-20% workers compensation insurances fees and may not realize how they drastically cut into the bottom line.

Let me explain how all of this works. A caregiver making $8.00 as a subcontractor only costs the agency $8.00 per hour and allows the agency to keep any additional reimbursement as profit.

By having to pay the extra 7.65% matching Social Security taxes the caregiver is making the equivalent of $7.31 an hour. In addition to making less, the caregiver also has no Worker Compensation Insurance and no Unemployment Insurance. Does this seem fair? Not to me. Nonetheless, it's a real part of the present day system, and you need to be aware of it.

Look how different the scenario is when these workers are properly classified as employees (which in virtually all of the cases, they are). A caregiver making $8.00 as an employee keeps the $8.00 while the employer covers the Workers Compensation, Unemployment Insurance, and Social Security. The actual cost to this agency is $9.69 to $10.49 per hour depending on the Workers Compensation rate, which fluctuates.

But, you may ask, is Workers Comp really that important? Well, let's revisit that accident that Jane had (falling in the shower) at the beginning of the chapter. For the sake of argument, let's assume that she has no Workers Compensation. Further, let's say she has $8,500 in medical bills and has been out work for three months now and has to seek compensation. She hires an attorney to go after the employer for the damages and the attorney advises her that since she was hurt working for you, you may also be liable. The attorney finds out you own your home and decides to sue for the value of your home for damages. That sickening feeling you had when Jane was injured has now gotten even worse.

Does this sound far fetched? Well, it's not. In fact, this is a very real scenario and happens to people just like you every day on a daily basis. Don't take risks, educate yourself and protect yourself from the ignorance bug. Detailed information can be found in the IRS Publication 15-A and your state's insurance code.

But there's more to a good agency than just taking care of Social Security and Workers Comp. If Jane works for a really good agency, she will also have other benefits. Health Insurance is the most important of these. In fact, many workers will stay on the job simply to maintain their health insurance coverage. That means she is more likely to stick with her job rather than leave and seek greener pastures. And job retention is a critically important issue, not only for the caregivers themselves, but also for the person receiving care. When the same person or group of people is taking care of you year after year, you build up a rapport and often even strong friendships. This is so vital to the disabled, invigorating both their minds and bodies as they cope with the challenges of daily living. Of course, health insurance is expensive, and, sadly, you will find very few agencies willing to go this extra step. However, such agencies are indeed out there. You just have to spend the time and energy to search for them. Like your mother always said, Do your homework!

The bottom line is this: Make sure your caregivers are paid professionally and are taken care of so they can better taken care of you. A happy employee, treated fairly with dignity and respect, will not only stay on the job longer, he or she in all likelihood will also do a *better* job. And isn't that what it's all about, quality care? That's why I think other benefits, in addition to Health Insurance and Workers Comp, are so important. One of the most vital, in my opinion, is paid vacation time. Imagine working all year without a vacation! We all need a break, especially people working in high stress, low pay jobs such as taking care of the disabled. Getting a chance to kick back for a week or so to recharge the old batteries is a good thing for all of us. Think how grateful the employee will be when he comes back to work fresh and relaxed. You might also want to offer the option of exchanging part of the employee's paid vacation time for cash. In other words, the caregiver only takes part of his vacation time but gets paid for the unused portion. That may not seem like a million bucks. And to you or I it might not mean that much. But for an overstressed worker in an under-appreciated field, it just might mean everything.

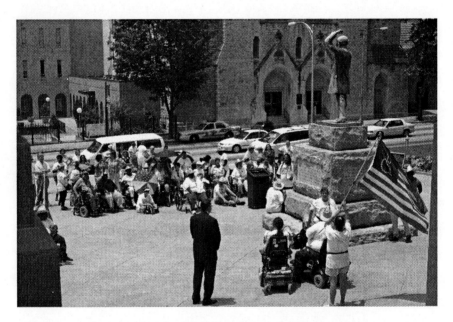

speaking with the politicians after the parade

NOTES:

<u>NOTES</u>

Chapter Four
Staffing and Interviewing
your Caregivers

Now that you've decided to use a staffing or employee leasing service, it's time to get into more detail. How exactly does it work? Let's start at the beginning. Conducting interviews. A staff service will meet with you and interview you to find out what your needs are so they can interview potential employees on your behalf. Or, if you prefer, you can let them know that you prefer to conduct the interviews yourself. With an employee leasing service, in fact, they will require that you do the interviewing yourself. That's OK, because I think taking this crucial matter into your own hands is a good idea. When you see how the interviewing process works, you will understand why.

Before we begin, let me offer you an important tip. When you are arranging for a potential employee to come in to meet you for the first time, don't refer to your meeting as an interview. Just tell the applicant you would like to "meet them." Why do I suggest this? I have found if you tell a caregiver they have to go through an interview, immediately they begin to feel intimidated. In fact, from my experience I know that only about 2 out of every 10 people you schedule for an interview will actually show up. Many of these people, having only worked low wage jobs all of their lives, lack confidence and suffer from low professional self-esteem. They end up talking themselves out of seizing the initiative and going on the interview. If you call it a meeting, the number of no shows declines to about 50%.

This reluctance to face an interview, when you think about it, does make a certain amount of sense. We all know how much pressure there can be when going on a job interview. Sometimes you agonize about it for days ahead of time. You start to feel the pressure of having to "perform" well at the interview. You begin to worry about the competition and what you can say or do that will give you an edge. Spare your potential caregivers all of these headaches. Keep it simple and informal. That way there will be less pressure on the applicants and they won't feel like they are under the gun. It might also create a better atmosphere for you to get a good feeling for just exactly who this person is, and what it is that makes him or her tick. At a formal interview, people tend to keep their guard up. They may be more likely to "be themselves" in this more informal setting and without so much pressure.

Of course, in reality it really is an interview. Be prepared. First of all, it's a good idea to have the agency do some pre-screening well before you even meet any of the prospective caregivers. This can be as extensive as you want it to be, and you can tailor it to your own needs. For example, you can tell the agency that you want somebody over 18 or over 25. Here's why those particular ages are important. Workers under age 18 will have certain restrictions because they are minors. As for being under 25, that makes a difference when it comes to your car insurance. There is an added surcharge for drivers under 25, and you may need the caregiver to use your vehicle for grocery shopping or other tasks, which means you will need to add this person to your insurance. I know of one gentleman who employs eight girls to help with his care. All of them sometimes have to drive his van, so he had to add all eight of their names to his insurance policy.

The prescreening process can go well beyond these simple basics. You can also ask the agency to do drug screening on the applicants, as well as a background check to see if they have a criminal record. Furthermore, if they're going to be driving your car, you will want to be sure to have the agency pull their driving record from the Department of Motor Vehicles (DMV).

Let me also point out that, if you're not working with an agency, you can still enjoy the comfort and security provided by a criminal background check. Simply ask the applicants to bring the background check themselves, which they can get from the local sheriff's office. You may also want them to bring along documentation (if they have it) showing that they have been trained in CPR and First Aid.

When it's finally time to start meeting with the people the agency sends to you, be sure to know well in advance the questions that you want to ask. You may want to take notes as you go along, but try to do it in an unobtrusive sort of way. In other words, don't be writing away furiously in a notebook as the applicant responds to each question. Try to reserve the note taking only for certain key points you want to be sure to remember, and do so in a somewhat relaxed and casual manner.

I strongly suggest that you get personal with the applicants. Make them feel at home (after all, you'll probably be interviewing them in the very same house where they will be working). Don't pre judge any of the people you meet with by their initial appearance.

Maybe they are overweight. Maybe they aren't dressed well (sweat pants and a T shirt, for example). Maybe they seem, at least from their outward appearance, not like the kind of person you would want to hire to work in your place of business. Well, that's OK because they're *not* going to be working in a business environment, they're going to be working in your home. It won't really matter how they dress. The kind of work they will be doing will involve things such as cleaning and household chores and helping a disabled person with the tasks of daily living and personal issues. That person who may at first glance appear somewhat slovenly may, in fact, turn out to be the perfect candidate. The old cliché about not being able to judge a book by its cover really is true, so wait until after you speak with this person until you form your opinions.

It usually makes sense to begin with some of the obvious background questions. Ask about their work history. Have they ever done this kind of work before? Don't be surprised if many of them answer no. However, an individual's lack of experience or training shouldn't necessarily exclude her from consideration for the job. Keep in mind that the character and personality of the individual is what you really need to focus on. You can train a decent, easy- going person to be a good worker. But if you have a person of low character, even if he or she has some prior training or experience, would this really be somebody you want working in your home? Ask yourself, does this seem like somebody I can trust, someone I can rely on? If the answer is no, you need to keep searching.

There are a number of other questions you should be sure to ask. Try to find out a little bit more about the person by asking questions that don't directly relate to the job. For example, what kinds of hobbies or interests does she have? A sports fan? Which teams? Is she from this area? Does she have any plans for the future? Remember, don't turn it into an interrogation. Make it more like a friendly conversation between two people just getting to know each other. To help break the ice, offer some personal information about yourself, perhaps telling the applicant a bit about your own background. Don't necessarily focus only on your disability and the specific kind of assistance you will require. That can all be explained later. For now, keep it informal. The more you loosen up, the person seeking the job will too.

Just be sure not to get *too* personal. I want you to realize that when it comes to hiring employees these days, there are all sorts of rules and regulations regarding what you can and cannot ask. For example, you can't ask the person their age or marital status. Still, there are ways around these limitations. The more you engage in conversation, the more information will indirectly come your way. You may well end up finding out, for example, whether or not the applicant has kids. People love to talk about their kids and most parents will inevitably end up telling you about them. They may even not be able to resist showing you pictures (especially if you have kids and you bring up the subject first).

So what do you do with all of that information you've been able to glean? Use it to your advantage! For example, maybe you've discovered that the woman you've been talking to is a single mom. Does that disqualify her? Absolutely not. However, be realistic and don't be afraid to ask some probing questions. Let's face it, having kids means there will be many occasions when the caregiver will not be able to come into work. It may be because one of the kids is sick, there is some event at school, it could be school vacation week, etc. There are hundreds of possibilities. It is fair for you to ask what kind of a plan would she have in place to handle these contingencles. It may well be that she has an excellent support system, perhaps close friends or family members who can step in and help her with the kids while she is at work. That would be great. Of course, if she has no way of covering when she has a "kid problem," it's OK for you to let this influence your decision when it comes to hiring.

You should also be certain to find out what their transportation situation is like. How far away from your home does this person live? Does she own a car? If the answer is yes, don't make the assumption that that necessarily is a positive thing. Think about it, if it's an old car, it might break down every other week. And if it's snowy, she might be late or not even be able to come in because of the sloppy roads (or an unplowed driveway). Actually, it might be better if the caregiver needs to rely on public transportation such as buses or trains. These methods of transportation are extremely reliable and can deposit her at your front door right on schedule in almost any weather. So carefully consider the answer you receive when you ask that vital question about commuting.

Finally, be sure that before your meeting ends you have given the applicant a thorough understanding of what precisely the job entails and what will be expected of her on a daily basis. Encourage the people you meet with to ask questions. Make sure they know exactly what they're getting into. Otherwise, you might end up hiring this person and a few weeks into the job she is shocked to find out what some of her duties are. Then she quits. And you have to start the whole process over again. It's better to be up front about every detail you can think of. Honesty is always the best policy. You will never regret it.

Then there is the bottom line: money. Don't even discuss this topic until you have finished with everything else. But don't try to avoid it either. After all, it is a job that you are offering and people apply for a job in order to make money. Tell them very forthrightly what you are willing to pay and ask if the amount falls into their range. They will always want more, of course, but most of them will never say it, at least not at this stage. For your part, as I said, be forthright, BUT, as in any negotiation, never give away your top price right at the beginning! Let's say I know that the top amount I can afford to pay a caregiver is $8 per hour. Well, you can bet that during our initial meeting I'm not going to tell the applicant that she will be starting (if hired) at $8 per hour. I suggest you say something like this. "We can have you start at $6.50 an hour, and if things work out after a 30 day trial period, your pay will go up by 50 cents an hour." By saying that you will be accomplishing two things. First, you won't be locking yourself into a higher pay scale right from the beginning, with a person you don't even know very well yet. Second, you will be establishing within the prospective employee's mind the notion that her wages will be directly related to her performance. It never hurts to start driving that concept home right from the start. Of course, you have to stick to your end of the bargain too. Clearly explain to this person that if you hire her and she does a good job for you, there will be a raise (of roughly 25 cents per hour) every few months, after a job performance review. Sometimes the agency will provide you with such a review, and if they do you should request that in be in writing rather than verbal. And if you are going to be offering any sorts of benefits with the job (including but not limited to vacation time and personal time) right now is your opportunity to thoroughly discuss how that will work and to answer any questions about it.

Always keep in mind that hiring people, and the overall employer / employee relationship, is a two way street. If you want to be treated with dignity and respect (remember, the person you hire will by necessity become involved with some highly personal issues with you), be sure that you show that same kind of dignity and respect to your prospective caregiver. That's the best way to successfully set the stage for what will hopefully become a rewarding experience for both of you.

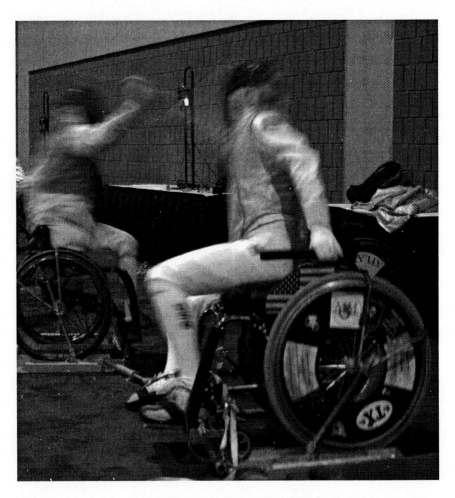

Fencing at the Atlanta Nationals

<u>NOTES</u>

<u>NOTES</u>

Chapter Five
Problem Solving and
Effective Communication

We all know that sometimes we can be our own worst enemy. Everything may be going along like smooth sailing....until we do something to torpedo our own ship! Well, the same is true when it comes to hiring competent people to assist either yourself or a loved one who requires in home care. That's why I can't overstate how important it is not to *create your own problems*.

Now, I can almost hear some of you saying as you read those words, "What is he talking about? I would never do anything that would hurt myself." No, not intentionally. But even little oversights can sometimes lead to big problems. Let me give you an example. Let's say we have a person who requires care. This person also requires certain medications that he is supposed to take every day. What if he forgets to take the medication? Yes, it will have a negative effect on his health, and that's bad enough. It may also, however, have unforeseen consequences for the caregiver. Missing certain medications can lead to side effects that often include mood swings and changes in sleep habits. Just think for a moment how much added stress that can put on the caregiver. It may be that as part of her job the caregiver expected that this person would be asleep for much of her shift. Now, because of missing his medication, he is wide awake and in need of attention. Maybe not a huge problem…unless, for example, the caregiver happened to be a student (as many of them are) and was planning on using that "sleep time" as an opportunity to study for important exams. It's especially frustrating because this is a situation that could have easily been avoided simply by taking the proper medicines as prescribed.

The consequences could be even worse. There are certain drugs that doctors prescribe because they help with an individual's state of mind. Not taking these medications as instructed can frequently lead to drastic mood swings. A person may become grouchy, irritable, hyperactive, etc. Generally, he becomes a nightmare to be around, let alone try to take care of. Yet again, this was a completely avoidable situation, if only the person receiving care would exercise some responsibility when it comes to taking his medications.

The rate of turnover in the caregiver profession is already too high. Irresponsible behavior on the part of those they are taking care of will inevitably lead to even higher turnover. Make sure this doesn't happen with your caregiver. Especially if she is a person whom you really have come to know, trust and like. It would be a real tragedy to throw away a good thing so needlessly.

Let me show you another example of how a caregiver could easily become disillusioned with her job. I've seen many cases where people try to *micromanage* their caregivers. A very common, yet telling example involves something as mundane as your laundry. "C'mon," you say, "what kind of controversy could there be over laundry?" You might be surprised. We all get used to doing things our own way. Let's say we have an elderly woman who has been doing her own laundry for seventy years. For all those years, as far back as she can remember, she always did it in a very specific way. She has a special non-allergic detergent that she uses. OK, that would be easy enough for the caregiver. But what if she also had specific directions, down to the smallest, most insignificant details, of where the detergent cup goes when finished, exactly how much detergent to use, what corner of the laundry room it needs to be stored in, etc. It could get pretty maddening for the person trying to keep up with all of that and do every little thing "just the right way."

Don't think that I'm exaggerating, either. I know of a real life person who did all of the above. And a whole lot more. The laundry room was only the beginning of her choreography. It extended throughout the entire house. She would even instruct the caregivers as to the exact positioning of a pill bottle on the counter. It had to be precisely one inch from the edge. The laundry, not surprisingly, also required a carefully choreographed production. The poor girl who worked for her had to put each article of clothing into the wash machine in a painstakingly calculated order. It had to be first this shirt, then these pants, then these socks, etc. They then had to be removed from the dryer the exact same way! Predictably, three caregivers came and went within days of each other. They didn't even bother to call to quit, they just bolted as quickly as they could to escape her aggravating demands. One of the caregivers finally stayed long enough to tell us what was going on. Soon afterwards, she quit too. The real shame of this situation was that she was otherwise such a nice elderly lady. Even the caregivers thought so. But her obsessive micromanaging of virtually everything in her house was just too much for them to take.

The opposite of micromanaging, of course, is to be completely disorganized. This extreme is not a good idea either. Yes, you are the one receiving care. However, that does not mean that you are helpless and don't need to pitch in. Quite to the contrary. You can make a huge contribution by simply doing some common sense planning ahead of time. It is also a great way to show that you are respectful of your caregiver. This person, remember, is doing a tough job for low pay. Wouldn't it be the right thing to do to make her job a bit easier? An example would be to make sure that when the caregiver goes to store you make a comprehensive list of all of the items she needs to pick up. It's really not fair to make her have to go all the way back to the store because there was something you carelessly forgot. By staying organized and planning ahead, it just makes everyone's life run more smoothly.

However, being well organized doesn't mean there will never be arguments. They are inevitable in all human relationships. Still, people receiving care have a responsibility (as does the caregiver) to do all they can to limit conflicts. Have you ever noticed that most conflicts are created when people have too much time on their hands? Sitting around all day doing nothing, even if you have a severe disability, is never a good thing. Maybe it's on a subconscious level, but somehow people inevitably end up causing problems when there is nothing to keep their minds occupied. That's why keeping busy is so vital (not to mention the health benefits). Regardless of age or disability there are groups out there that have all sorts of activities people can get involved with. I suggest you contact the YMCA or AARP for more information.

Make sure you understand the way things work today. Don't think it is like the "olden days" anymore. These days, there are sports for the disabled such as tennis, swimming and many others. You can also get involved with non sports related activities to keep you busy, including things like Bingo (a favorite amongst the elderly), church activities and attending plays and musical performances. The possibilities are endless when you really put your mind to it.

It is crucial that you get friends and relatives involved. Have fun with them rather than always just asking them to help you out with stuff. Spending time with a disabled or elderly person doesn't have to be a "chore" at all. To the contrary, it can be a fun time that both parties look forward to.

Put away the excuses for sitting around doing nothing! With just a little bit of research you will find that there are many groups that empower people to become more active with things such as fencing, scuba, arts and crafts, and horseback riding. They often have programs that are specifically designed to take into account the participants' age and / or disability. There are also games such as checkers and chess, as well as online chat groups, which are increasingly popular today. One of these groups that does a fine job empowering people to become more active is Endeavor Freedom, located here in Georgia. We do all sorts of activities. Through this group a good friend of mine, who happens to be disabled, has become a member of the National Fencing Team.

Here are some more ways to avoid problems. Be sure to always treat your employees fairly. A good step in this direction would be giving them holidays off (with pay) if this is possible. Try to look at things from their point of view as best as you are able. For example, let them know everything (all of the day to day tasks) that needs to be done well ahead of time so they can pace themselves. That's so much better than giving them each task one by one. At least this way they feel like they're making progress. Otherwise, the day begins to seem endless. They start feeling like they can never get a break. Would you like a work environment like that? Of course not, so extend to them the same courtesy you would want for yourself.

Above all, be sure to always treat caregivers professionally. It's a sad fact that many homebound people do not get out much and can wrongly direct sexual behavior toward a caregiver. This cannot be tolerated. Such behavior toward an employee constitutes sexual harassment and is against the law. This is not so much a problem with the elderly, but happens quite a bit with younger people who are disabled. With the elderly it tends to be more of a somewhat harmless flirtation, but it is still something that should be avoided.

Another problem you can take proactive steps to avoid involves the employee's salary. That's why it is vital that you choose an agency that processes their payroll in a prompt manner so employees get paid on time. Believe me, there is nothing that will cause more problems than a late paycheck. It may even make the caregiver quit, especially if it happens more than once. And who could blame them, especially when they are already making low wages to begin with. Even worse, having to wait for that paycheck could really mess up the caregiver's budget by making her bills late, which could damage her credit rating as well. So pay careful attention to see if your caregiver is having a problem with this. If so, tell her you are going to straighten it out right away. Call the agency and tell them they need to fix this problem immediately.

If not, you will take your business elsewhere. That usually is all it takes.

I recommend that you provide written reviews for your caregivers every three months to keep the lines of communications open regarding job expectations and the results that you've observed. Are they on time, late, missing days, getting everything done? You should also solicit feedback regarding your relationship with them. Is the way they're being instructed working? Is communication working? Do they need a list of tasks? Written instructions? Are there any problems? Also, if they are always on time and doing a good job, this is your opportunity to give them some praise. When a person isn't making a lot of money, a little appreciation goes a long way.

Remember, always take the caregiver's point of view into consideration, as they may very well have quite justified concerns. Let's say an employee is always at the workplace (the home where the disabled person lives) 15 minutes late (9:15 in the morning). Don't jump to the conclusion that she is lazy or doesn't care about punctuality. Did you ever think there might be a legitimate reason? Maybe she has to drive through a badly congested traffic area. As we all know, traffic is unpredictable. So leaving an extra 15 minutes early might not be the solution. If she leaves 15 minutes early, and there is no traffic, then she will be there well before her shift starts, which is not really fair to her. Perhaps you could offer an alternative: change her schedule to 10:00, well after the traffic has subsided, or accommodate her in some other way. The point is, don't just blame her! Get to the root of the problem and then, together and in the spirit of cooperation, work to solve it.

Finally, when hiring employees be sure to be very specific about job expectations and draw out exactly what they are being hired for. This way it will be perfectly clear to both parties what is expected of them and will alleviate many potential problems before they ever start. After all, the best way to solve a problem is to keep it from happening in the first place.

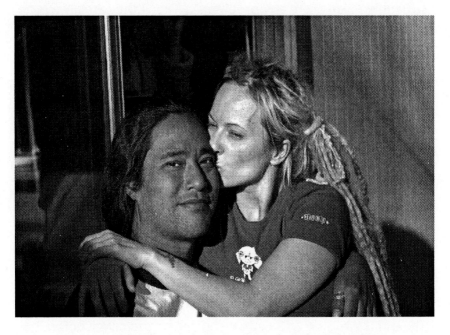

Zen gets a thank you from Tanja at her Birthday Party.

<u>NOTES</u>

<u>NOTES</u>

Chapter Six
Daily routine and scheduling

Are you an organized person? Maybe you are, maybe not. However, if you are going to have caregivers helping you with the tasks of daily living, I want to strongly encourage you to become as organized as possible. No, that doesn't mean transforming into some sort of robot that does everything the same way all the time. I realize and appreciate that variety is the spice of life. But it's in your own best interests to have a certain amount of orderliness in your daily routine. It will make life so much easier for your caregiver, which will have the ripple effect of making life better for you too.

Think about it for a moment. Imagine going to your job every day and never knowing what to expect. Your boss changes your tasks, the order you do them in, and just about everything else whenever he feels like it. Not exactly the ideal work environment, right? But that's exactly what you're subjecting your caregiver to if you do not formulate a detailed schedule for her, one that fits in well with your own needs and activities. She will be doing one thing today, something else tomorrow and then switch all over again the day after that. I can tell you with almost near certainty that she will burn out really fast under those circumstances.

There is a better way. Make a plan…then stick to it. Yes, of course you can make changes whenever necessary. Just be sure to first take into consideration the effect your change will have on those around you, especially your caregivers.

The best way to make a plan is to be proactive and start the process before you even hire a caregiver. A good place to begin is by keeping a journal. I suggest that you keep track of your daily activities (your routine) for at least one full week. That way you will include both weekdays and weekend days, which may vary significantly from one another. Your journal will be an excellent tool for gauging just what exactly it is you do every day, and when you do it.

Start with when you wake up and what you do first. These are the kinds of things that can differ so much from one person to the next. Do you like to take a shower right away, or is that something that you prefer to do later in the day? Do you eat a large breakfast (or do you skip it altogether?). These questions and many more need to be answered in as much detail as possible. Make sure you write down every detail of your day, when you do it, and how long it takes. If possible keep track of any reasons *why* you do something at a certain time; this will be helpful later on when you work on prioritizing your day.

Now, how does all of this affect your caregiver? For starters, the reason why you do certain things at certain times may be precisely because you need the assistance of a caregiver. For example, perhaps there is a particular time of day that you bathe. If you require assistance with this, make sure that the caregiver understands this activity will be one of her daily tasks and it will normally be at 7:00 every other night. You should be sure to carefully distinguish in your journal those tasks that you feel comfortable doing on your own and those you need assistance with. In this way your caregiver will be much better prepared for each workday.

The next step comes after you have faithfully recorded all of your activities in your journal for a period of seven to thirty days. Why so long? A month will give you a good idea of your full routines. This may include things that would otherwise be overlooked such as doctor's appointments, shopping trips, etc.

I want to emphasize the importance of not forgetting the small details (because they are indeed so easy to forget!). For example, what about food? Do you need to have a cooked lunch? Who cooks it? What about dinner? Also, are there certain days when you need to be someplace? Maybe it is a Bingo game, or some sort of activity at an elderly center. Will the caregiver need to drive you there? All of the different things that comprise your daily living need to be taken into account. Keep that pencil nearby. You may be surprised at how often you need to make journal entries.

OK, you've now been keeping the journal for a month. The next step is to go back over it and carefully match up those things for which you need assistance, with how much time it will take you to accomplish each one of them (with help), and then you will be able to prioritize what your needs are. What do I mean by prioritization, and why is it so important? Prioritizing means figuring out which things you do every day really are essential. It means figuring out if you really need help with those things, or can you do them on your own, only more slowly. The answers will have a huge impact on your budget. It will even help answer the very fundamental question of home health care, is it feasible and safe for you.

By using your meticulously recorded journal, you will see exactly what you need assistance with, and what you can do on your own. How many hours of help do you need every week? The answer, of course, will have to be based on how much you can afford. Let's say one hour per week is all you can afford; then it's not safe. Clearly, for a person who needs assistance that would not be nearly enough time. It would mean you are cutting corners to save money, but very possibly putting your safety in jeopardy in the process. Fortunately, there are few people whose financial circumstances are so dire as to allow only one hour per week of assistance.

A more realistic scenario might be that you can afford 12 hours per week. In some cases, that may actually be too many hours. You may be an elderly person who simply needs some help with house cleaning and other routine household duties. In such a case, five hours per week might be sufficient. Again, your journal is the key. It is a way to make it an organized decision. It will help you describe the job when you contact an agency or write up an ad.

Being so well organized will pay huge dividends when you finally are ready to make a job offer and hire a caregiver. It's a good idea to have a meeting with your prospective new caregiver to go over, in detail, what a typical day is like for you. Don't hold anything back. It's best to be up front with this new helper so she can know exactly what her job will entail. This will let her make an informed decision whether or not she wants to accept the job. After all, not only would it be dishonest to hide any of the details, but if your day is filled with too many tasks for her she will obviously find that out soon enough…and then it will be back to the drawing board for you as you start the hiring process all over again. Don't make it sound overwhelming, of course. Let the caregiver know that you are a reasonable person and you try to never be too demanding. But if the day is going to be busy, make sure you're hiring a hard worker who will not find it too strenuous and will quit not long after starting.

Once your new person has accepted the job, you need to be sure to create a schedule of when things need to be done around your house. For example, vacuum on Thursdays (at a certain time) or bathe at 9 am so you can make your water aerobics class at eleven. You get the idea. Very hands on, practical, everyday sorts of things. The more detail the better. We want to make the schedule as unambiguous as possible. Even if you find a subject a bit touchy or sensitive, bring it up anyway. For example, do you have bathroom needs? If so, make sure your caregiver knows about it.

I'll let you in on a little secret. One place where many people go wrong with scheduling is they do an excellent job of planning out each individual day, but they lose sight of the big picture. In other words, they have their typical day planned out, but not their entire week. And during a week, there may be activities and tasks that are not part of every day. For example, medical appointments. Make sure your schedule includes all your appointments to reduce surprises. There is nothing worse for a caregiver than getting all their tasks finished and thinking they are about to get a little break only to find out they have to rush off to get you to a doctor appointment that you neglected to mention. Caregivers do not make enough for what they do and anything that makes their day go more smoothly will allow you to get better care. Remember, the old saying, "what goes around comes around," is a very basic fact of life.

There are certain tasks that come up on a regular basis that some people assign to their caregivers that need to be clearly written into the schedule. They may be things that need to be done every week, such as taking out the trash. Or it might be every few weeks, such as mowing the lawn. Other things may only need to be taken care of once per month. Paying bills would be a good example. As a general rule, I don't think you should have your caregiver pay your bills (I don't mean provide the money, I mean write out the checks, envelopes, etc.). It's not a good idea to ask them to get involved with your private money matters and business. However, if you are physically incapable of bill paying, you may want to ask the caregiver to help out with this monthly chore. If you do, be sure the bills are well organized. It would be a real added burden on the caregiver if, because of your mismanagement, she messed up your bills and caused you financial problems. She'd feel guilty, you'd be angry. Not a good scene. It can be avoided through proper organization.

In fact, organization is so important that I recommend you conduct an organization overview. You may think you have all of your bases covered, but do you really? What about when things go wrong? You know what they say about the "best laid plans of mice and men…" They always go astray. You can never predict what the future will bring. Neither can your caregiver. But life will be so much easier for both of you if, in addition to being well organized, you also have a workable, realistic contingency plan for when things go wrong (because you know, as we all do, that inevitably they will).

When you are already well organized, making a contingency plan is really not all that hard. You will even find that emergencies (or potential emergencies) truly bring out the strength of your organizational skills. Being organized means less headaches, and that's something that all of us can appreciate.

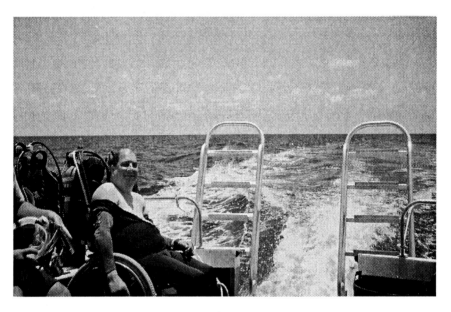

Tony Relaxing after a great dive in the Bahamas

NOTES

Chapter Seven
Plan of Care and Putting It To Use

In the previous chapter we discussed the importance of having a schedule and the necessity of sticking to it. We saw that the various rhythms of your daily routine have a significant impact on your caregiver, making her job much easier if the two of you are on the same page. But you need more than just a workable schedule. You also need a plan of care. Think of it as a blueprint for both you and your caregiver, setting out the goals you have in mind by receiving in-home care. In other words, once you and your caregiver clearly understand what you hope to accomplish, it will be much more likely that you will achieve it.

A plan picks up where your schedule leaves off. It actually goes beyond a schedule because it includes goals. And goals make more of a difference than you may have realized when it comes to receiving assistance from a caregiver. They provide direction for both of you, which can make each day more focused and meaningful.

Now, the particular goals that you are aiming for will vary from one individual to another. It begins with asking yourself the question, "Why do I need care in the first place?" The answer often has to do with something that you have been having difficulty with. For example, a goal could to stay independent and continue living at home. For various health reasons (either from a disability or advancing age) maintaining that independence has become more difficult for you. You can't do for yourself all of the things you once took for granted. But you know that with just the right amount of help you can still live in your own home and remain independent. Therefore, that becomes your plan; it is what you are striving for, the goal you are hoping to achieve.

Be sure to break the larger overall goal (i.e., maintaining your current lifestyle) into smaller, incremental milestones that you can attain within a reasonable amount of time – in fact, making a little progress every day. For example, an elderly person who is concerned about not getting enough exercise can set as a goal, "Get myself to where I walk every day." Or if the concern is spending too much time sitting around the house, the goal may be to join an activities group and attend as often as possible.

Most people receiving in-home care (except in certain cases such as a person recovering from an automobile accident) aren't going to get better. For example, if they currently walk a mile a week, they probably won't ever be able to walk two. On the other hand, they don't want things to get worse. So their goal could be to simply maintain the lifestyle they already have. Make sure they keep walking that mile, for instance. That would be a realistic goal because it is achievable. Every day that person gets out and walks a certain distance, he will have a feeling of accomplishment. He has succeeded in what he set out to do. And that is vital to one's mental health, as well as their physical well-being.

For a younger or middle-aged person dealing with a disability, the goal could be going back to college or taking adult education classes. The caregiver would provide the extra help to get them ready for their classes. If he's a painter, for example, the caregiver could help set up the paints and art equipment for his projects at home. This student's long term goals would have concrete results as he attends class each day, completes each course, and especially if he eventually receives a degree. For a disabled person struggling with life's difficulties, achieving such a goal can bring tremendous satisfaction, a sense of victory despite the obstacles.

Your plan of care should be revised regularly. As we all know, everything in our lives changes over time. An excellent opportunity to review and revise your plan of care is when you are conducting your employee review. All of the information regarding your care at that point will be fresh and updated. You will also want to be sure to get input and feedback from your caregiver. This is when both of you, together, can evaluate what is working, and what is not working. Anything that is going wrong can at this point be adjusted and corrected. Let's say, for instance, that you take a shower every morning at nine. But it always seems to take longer than expected and you keep missing an appointment. Well, that's a clear signal that you need to make a change. Perhaps it might be a good idea to instead shower the night before.

A plan of care doesn't have to be an exhaustive document. In fact, it should only be about two pages, one with your schedule and one with your goals and what you are hoping to achieve. Again, these goals are not to run a marathon or climb a mountain. Rather, they will be practical, attainable things such as being able to live at home for five more years (at a bare minimum) as an independent member of the community. Now that's something that is both realistic and achievable, and you can have a certain measure of success with it every day.

Schedule your day from morning till night and create a plan outlining the best ways and time to get things done. Those incremental goals I mentioned make all the difference in the world. Something that will take a year or more may well seem too daunting, too remote. But when a person can see a little bit of progress on a daily basis, they stay motivated. They stay focused.

Think about it. If you were planning on driving across the country, when you look at a map of the United States and see those 3,000 miles from sea to shining sea it may look like a long, arduous journey. However, if you break the trip into smaller segments, realizing the distance you will cover each day and the many states you will visit along the way, the map (at least in your mind) begins to shrink. That is why big, long term goals, are more easily digestible when you break them down into their individual components where you can feel like you are accomplishing something every day.

I recommend that you create and store your plan in a computer, if possible, so that frequent changes and fine-tuning can be made. The computer will also make sure the plan does not get lost (especially if you keep a back-up copy on a disc in a safe place). Keep a printed copy at all times so you can refer back to it whenever necessary. It should also include all of your medications and when you need to be taking them, as well as any appointments you have, especially doctor appointments. This printout should be the first thing a caregiver reads when she starts working for you, as it summarizes everything she will need to know. Remember, as I said, it's important for both of you to be on the same page.

In the Plan of Care a third page can be added, which I highly recommend. This would be an emergency action page. It should include your Name, Address, Phone Number, Health Insurance Information, Doctor's name and contact info, Hospital contact and location info., and Emergency contacts (i.e., family member or friend). It is also a good idea to list what actions to take in an emergency. For example, what should the caregiver do if the power goes out and you rely on a ventilator to breathe? How long will the battery last and is there an alternate power source? Knowing the answers to these questions could literally be a matter of life or death. So it is obviously well worth it to take just a few minutes and clearly spell out the proper instructions.

Let me share with you an experience that vividly illustrates the importance of being well prepared (there's a good reason why "Be Prepared" is the motto of the Boy Scouts). I once had a client who was on a ventilator. During a thunderstorm, a tornado was spawned. It roared into town and slammed into her home. She survived, even though a tree fell right into her room. However, the power was knocked out, threatening her life because the ventilator was about to shut down. Her caregiver went outside to start the generator…and was shocked to find that it didn't work! It had been sitting there for eight years, but had never been properly cared for. It was in a bad state of disrepair and this was no time to call for a repairman. Thankfully, firefighters came to the rescue and there was a happy ending. The Discovery Channel even did a show about this unfortunate incident. But the lesson about preparedness is what is truly important. If she had a written contingency plan, some of that hair-raising danger could have been avoided.

The plan of care also needs to include a brief bio of who you are. No, this isn't some sort of memoir of your life that you're writing for publication. Rather it is just a paragraph or two briefly explaining who you are and why you need assistance to live at home. An example may be that you want to stay independent in your own community rather than living in a nursing home. This section should also detail what you hope to achieve while living at home, and (don't leave this part out!) how the caregiver can best help you to attain those goals. This will provide the guidance she needs to offer you the highest quality care possible…which, after all, is the point of hiring her in the first place.

A typical bio, for an elderly person, might read like this:

"My name is Agnes Smith. I am 82 years old. I was widowed five years ago when my husband, Robert, died. I own my own home where I have lived for the past 49 years. I do not have a severe physical handicap, but there are some household tasks that I can no longer handle myself and I need help with. For example, I still like to cook but I can't reach up into the pantry to get at all of the pans and ingredients. And I no longer have the strength to take out the garbage or lift the laundry basket in the washroom, so I will need some assistance with that too.

One of my goals is to be able to walk to the corner store every day. However, my eyesight is not so good anymore and I need someone to help me when I cross the street. I also have some minor hygiene issues (doing my hair, using the shower, etc.) that I need help with. The right person will need to be available three days a week, which will also include driving me to my twice a week Bingo game at church and occasional doctor appointments."

Just remember, as in the above example, be clear, concise and to the point. Your caregiver will appreciate the attention to detail you provide, and it will mean less surprises – and therefore less hardship – for both of you down the road.

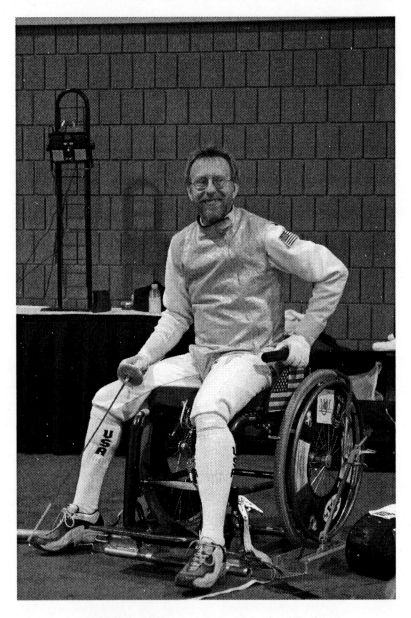

US National Fencer Gary Van der Wedge

<u>NOTES</u>

NOTES

Chapter Eight
Activities to get involved with

These days, being elderly or having a disability by no means implies that you are a "shut in" or a person who has no life outside of the house. To the contrary, today people of all ages and with all kinds of physical situations are more active than ever. What are they filling their days with? The list is almost endless. And the support system for these folks is vast, sophisticated and growing all the time. I will include a list of contact groups for elderly and disabled people at the end of this chapter.

When you think about, with so many good reasons for staying active – and so many opportunities – it's hard to imagine why anyone wouldn't take advantage of what's out there. The benefits make it well worth your while. Let's take a closer look at why keeping both your mind and body busy are so vital to your well being, both mentally and physically.

First of all, it will keep you busy. I can't think of anything worse than remaining inside my house 24 hours a day, 365 days a year. Talk about boring! That's no way to live, sitting around looking at the four walls all day. Not only will the muscles of your body begin to atrophy, your mind will become apathetic too. The more you are "out there" talking with people, exchanging ideas, living life to the fullest, the more you will feel a part of something greater than yourself. Something beyond just yourself. If you are disabled, it's good to also be amongst people without physical handicaps. You can learn from them and share in their experiences. For older people, it's always a good idea to get to know and be friends with people of all ages, including young people and kids (especially grandchildren). They can learn from your wisdom, and you can gain encouragement and a renewed zest for life from their vibrant youthfulness.

Furthermore, when you're engaged in fun and rewarding activities, it gives your life more of a sense of purpose. We all know that the disabled and the elderly share the same human dignity as the rest of us. However, a person can sometimes start feeling down on him or herself when they seem to have nothing to offer the outside world, nothing to contribute. Getting involved with activities is a great way to build up self-esteem and make you realize that you still have an important contribution to make to your community, and that you are still a vital player in the game called life. A sense of purpose can often keep us going even when things seem dark and bleak with tough times physically, or from the problems that inevitably tend to be a natural result of advanced aging.

The other benefit of staying active, of course, is the sheer fun and enjoyment of it, for both you and the person who is caring for you.

Sometimes, getting involved in activities can help maintain a connection with some things that were left behind as a result of a physical injury. For example, my good friend Zen Garcia, before the accident that resulted in his becoming quadriplegic, was into the Martial Arts in a big way. He had his Black Belt and many other impressive and notable achievements. Well, even though he is now quadriplegic, he refused to just give in to his disability and do nothing with his life. His interest in Martial Arts remained as strong as ever despite his new physical limitations. Rather than wallow in self-pity and do nothing about it, Zen opened himself up to new possibilities. Today, he is a proud member of the International Fencing Team. Once a week he goes to practice, and gives it his all. He is a true competitor, and he loves the challenge of overcoming whatever obstacles may stand in his way. He goes to tournaments and other fencing events. He has many friends through this participation, and it helps give a new sense of meaning and purpose to his life.

Now, something as intense as fencing may not be for you. But that's no excuse for not finding what IS right for you. As I said before, the list of potential activities is almost infinite. For starters, here's just a few random thoughts:

Ceramics

Bowling

Walking clubs

Pottery

Support Groups for your specific need

There are countless sporting events available

From my own experiences working with the elderly and disabled, I am well acquainted with many of the fine programs that exist today to serve our disabled and elderly citizens. In Atlanta, there are a number of organizations that have activities for disabled people. For example, I know that we have horseback riding, and I have seen it work wonders for those who have chosen to participate. I had a brain injured client who did this every week. It would be easy for people to assume that an individual with such a severe injury would not be able to handle an activity such as horseback riding. But nothing could be further from the truth. In fact, it provides a terrific outlet for pent up energy, a chance to get outside and enjoy the sights and sounds of nature, and it is something to look forward to every week. And that is just one of hundreds of examples I'm glad to report that I have personally become familiar with. Each program and, indeed, each individual; has their own inspiring stories that can encourage others in similar circumstances. Learn about them, and realize that you are not alone. Others have been where you are, they have traveled the very same path you now find yourself on. And they are enjoying life even though they may not be as physically able as they once were.

So where do you find all of these fun and rewarding activities? Do what everyone else does these days when they are seeking out information: turn to the Internet. For example, there is a fine website, www.disabilityresources.org that, as its name implies, provides valuable information for folks with disabilities. State parks are another excellent (often overlooked) resource. They have lots of programs with access for handicapped people.

As you delve into your research you will find that there are more classes for the elderly and disabled than you ever imagined.

Sailing classes, photography classes, bird watching, hikes, classes on botany, etc.. Some of it depends on where you live. So be sure to do that research. The more you look the more you will find.

But all the research in the world won't matter much if you take the information and then do nothing with it. The most critical part of getting involved with a new activity is to take that first step and actually do it. Lots of people come up with some wonderful ideas but then don't follow through with them. What a waste! I know sometimes it can be scary trying out something new for the first time. We all have a little apprehension about the unknown. It's perfectly normal. But you'll never find out what's on the other side of that door if you don't open it up and enter through it. There could be a whole world of possibilities just waiting for you, but nobody is going to make that first move. It has to be you.

Of course, as I touched on a moment ago, as you get involved with these activities you will quickly realize that you are not alone. There are many others out there living under the same circumstances as you. That is why it is best to get involved with a group and make a commitment. It will give you a sense of belonging, and the commitment will keep you from quitting if the going gets tough.

One last word about activities. Don't always think of just the obvious things, such as sports and hobbies. While these are great ideas, and I highly recommend them,. I also think you should use your imagination a bit. For example, volunteering your time and talent for worthy causes, such as charity work, may not be something that has crossed your mind. When you are elderly or disabled, the focus always seems to be on what can be done to help you. But you have so much to offer, there are so many ways that you can be the one who *provides* the help. Your participation will be greatly appreciated by those groups and organizations that need caring people such as you. There are telethons, fund-raisers and programs such as meals on wheels (yes, with the caregiver's help, I had a client who actually did this, serving those in need despite his own physical problems). Sometimes, giving back to the community in ways such as these can really boost your morale, and help you to maintain a healthy, active lifestyle. You look forward to waking up each morning when you have a mission to accomplish, and goals to achieve. And while it may be true that you need the help of others to get by in this world, it is just as true that there are others who need you.

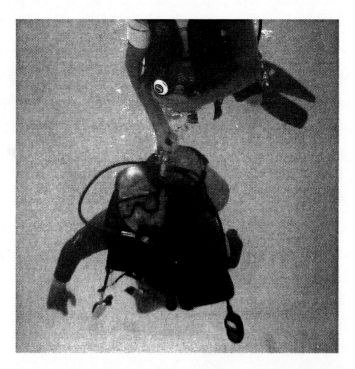

Tony heading down on our shark dive in the Bahamas.

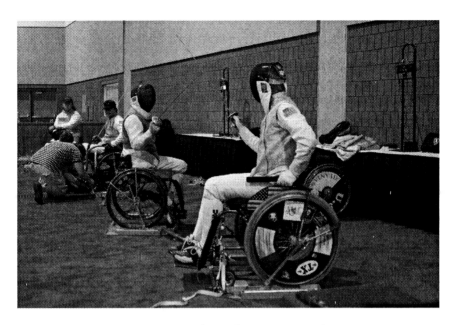

Fencing at the Atlanta Nationals

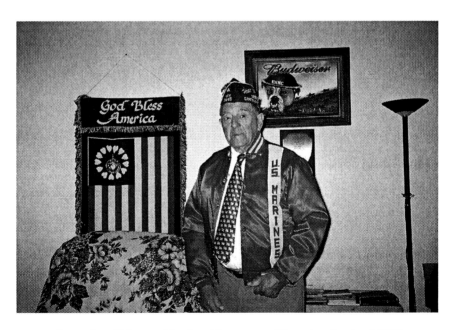

Grandpa Krieger Marine Veteran still active in the VFW

<u>NOTES</u>

Chapter Nine
Family Assistance

OK, by this point we have discussed many aspects of working with a caregiver. We've come to see how fundamental it is to find the right people, treat them well, and have an organized plan of care. However, even with the best caregivers in the world, it is still a great idea, if it is at all possible, to include family members and friends to help take care of you when you are at a point in life where you require assistance. This is a very important area because this kind of help really keeps things running smoothly. But it is also a somewhat sensitive subject. You know the old saying, "You always hurt the one you love." Well, I'm sure you're well aware that when it comes to asking family and friends for a helping hand, it can be easy for there to be a lack of good communications or misunderstandings. All of that can be avoided if you make an effort to approach the subject in the right way.

With caregivers being around so much of the time it is easy to get into the groove of just asking for everything you need. Since it's their job, you have the right to have certain expectations of them. After all, that is what they are being paid to do. However, you have no such rights when it comes to asking for things from friends and family. Remember, anything that they do for you is a favor, not an obligation. It is not their responsibility to take care of you. They are not paid caregivers.

Now, in all likelihood if you need assistance with something, those who are closest to you, your family and friends, probably will be more than willing to help. In fact, most people are glad to help out whenever they can and typically they will offer to do something without even being asked. Warning! Do not take advantage of this. Nobody owes you anything, so don't fool yourself into an "entitlement" mindset. This happens more frequently than you might realize, because when you are disabled or advanced in years it is easy to think, "I'm having a rough time of it, if they (family and friends) really cared they'd be doing more to help me." But this is not true. Simply by being born your kids did not sign up to be your caregiver for your life. And the fact that you have become sick or disabled does not obligate those around you to be at your beck and call. The best advice is to expect nothing and be grateful for all that you do receive. By the same token, when these folks help you, you owe them nothing in return. A simple yet heartfelt "thank you" should suffice.

I know from situations that I've seen over the years that people put too much of a load on family members. I remember a guy who would get on the phone and ask his family members for all kinds of things…all of the time. It was usually little stuff that could have waited until the caregiver got there. But rather than wait, he would always make it seem sort of urgent. So, wanting to help the guy, his friends and family would drop whatever they were doing and rush over to perform a simple task, run an errand, etc. After a while, however, they began to feel that they were being taken advantage of. Even his mother stopped coming over.

Visiting with him was one thing. Being his second string caregiver was quite another.

This situation occurs day in, day out in many families. It reminds me of the story about the little boy who cried wolf. Those around him grew wary of the false alarms, and when he really needed help, nobody was willing to come to his aid. The same thing happens when you call your friends and relatives up to come help out with every little thing. Save it for the big things that are absolutely necessary. Don't forget that, no matter how loyal and dedicated they may be to your comfort and well-being, they have their own lives to live too.

Of course, none of this is to imply that spending time with elderly or disabled people is some sort of a burden. To the contrary, I know from personal experience that it can be very enjoyable to hang out with my friends who have disabilities… yet they know the line not to cross with me because I have made it crystal clear to them. I do not mind, for example, grabbing a drink for a friend if his caregiver is not around. No problem. But it would be a problem if he expected to take it much further than that. For example, if you need assistance with getting into the shower or with relieving yourself, please don't ask friends or family to get involved, unless you know they are comfortable with it. Those are not the kinds of things they are going to be comfortable with, and it will make for quite an awkward situation. You are going to have to wait until one of the people trained to provide that sort of help arrives. I have made the line clear that I do not do anything "personal" because I am squeamish about that stuff.

You should assume that others will be squeamish too. Leave these personal care issues to the folks who are trained to do it. And are being paid for it. One of the best ways to lose a friend or alienate family members is to cross over that line. There may be no turning back. Other people may not so blunt as myself about drawing the line, but that too will lead to serious problems. Though they won't say it to your face, they may build up anger or resentment because you are always bugging them for stuff that can be done later by a paid employee, or perhaps it is something that you could go without for a little bit.

OK, how far does this concept go? Well, I certainly am not saying don't eat all day if, for instance, your caregiver is out sick and your sister is over. In this situation, you should feel free to ask if she could help out with lunch. My point is, just be appreciative of those around you for whatever help they offer. Never make any assumptions about what they can or should do for you. And remember, there are probably a number of things you can do for yourself, despite your physical limitations. Always make it a goal to personally take care of all responsibilities that you can handle by yourself.

Let me close this chapter with a few words about planning and scheduling. We covered these topics previously, but they become important when dealing with this issue of asking friends and family for assistance. Whatever you do, if you make plans with them, stick to those plans! Don't make last minute changes, and ask for the assistance that you will require as well in advance as possible. People lead incredibly busy lives these days, and while they may be kind hearted folks who want to help you, they won't appreciate it (to say the least) if you keep messing up their schedule and show little or no regard for how valuable their time is.

I will share a personal anecdote with you. I was going on a trip to Biloxi with a disabled friend of mine. I told him we would be ready to go at 1 pm on Saturday. Now, having been on many trips with him in the past I knew he would be late. Well, this time he was more than late. Saturday came and went, and no friend. Then on Sunday I finally heard from him, saying he was ready to go. By the time he showed up, I had had enough. How many times was I expected to put up with this? I decided not go. In fact, these days I rarely go on these kinds of trips anymore. I've been burned out by being stood up one too many times. This is no way to plan a trip or work with people who are going out of their way to get you somewhere! Yes (since I'm such a nice guy) I'm still friends with him, but I think you get the point. (By the way, the story did have a happy ending, When he finally showed up, he had a cute young woman with him. I decided to meet them in Biloxi after all…driving there on my own, of course!)

We all want to be treated with respect. We show respect to others by doing our best to stick with any scheduled plans we make, and to at least let them know if there has been a change in our plans. Having the assistance of friends and family can be one of the greatest blessing in life for a person who is disabled or elderly. Don't be too proud to accept their help. Go ahead and allow them to help you. Just don't take advantage of them. Have a grateful heart and be glad that they are good friends and true family.

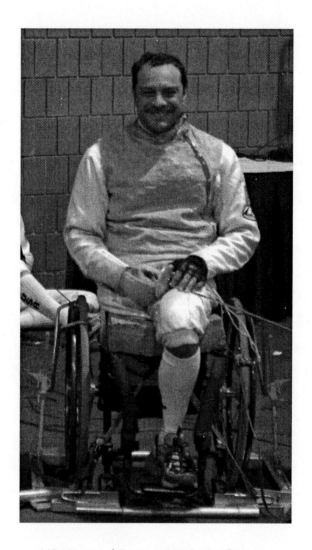

US National Fencer Mario Rodriguez

<u>NOTES</u>

NOTES

Chapter 10
Home Monitoring and Safety

We've now seen how many benefits there can be for the elderly and the handicapped by having someone there for them, right in their own home, to help them maintain their lifestyle and a very real sense of independent living. This can be a very valuable thing for not only the person who requires care, but for their friends and family as well. It's nice having others who can help share some of the duties of taking care of someone who needs assistance. However, as we've pointed out, there are going to be times when the people who are being cared for will still need to be left alone. How often this will happen will depend on how much care is required, and how many hours of care you can afford. In any case, be prepared for at least a certain amount of "alone time." This is a reality of the system.

But prepare how? you ask. By making sure that the home the person who requires care is living in provides as safe an environment as possible. I'm not suggesting that you turn it into a fortress, or that anyone be forced to live in some sort of "plastic bubble." But there are indeed a number of reasonable precautions that you need to be aware of. Most of them you can do yourself fairly easy and they are not too expensive. For starters, take into consideration who the person living in the home is and what potential dangers he or she may be facing. For example, if it is an elderly person (particularly if this individual suffers from Alzheimer's) chances are good that he or she is going to be forgetful about things. So you may want to make sure to render the stove inoperable before you leave for the day. The caregiver can do this very easily by switching off the fuse from the fuse box, if it's an electric stove, or turning off the gas for a gas stove. It's a better alternative than letting the poor soul turn on the stove, forget about doing it, and then burn the house down. Along these same lines, if the person can't drive you might want to take away the car keys. Imagine what a disaster could happen if her or she got behind the wheel. These steps will make the person that much more safer and will give those who love him some peace of mind.

Still, despite the best precautions, fires and other bad things can and do happen. You need to prepare ahead just in case the worst happens. Smoke alarms and carbon monoxide detectors are a must. But remember, they don't work if you don't consistently make sure they have fresh batteries. Change them in the spring and fall when you change your clocks. Or you may want to consider one of the hard wired models that run off of electricity…but still be sure to check the batteries periodically, they are used as a back-up in case there is a power failure.

There are other steps you can take to make the home a safer place. They are similar to what parents of young children do to "child proof" their homes. This is by no means to imply that an elderly or handicapped person is like a child, but the fact of the matter is, there comes a point in almost all of our lives when we need the assistance of other people to keep us safe. It is certainly not something to be ashamed of. You need to be sure that if there is a fire, for example, the person has the ability to get out of the house. If the person is alone and in a wheelchair, what would happen? First, it's a good idea to be sure the bedroom is on the first floor. Just as importantly, make sure there is a clear path to get out of the house if there is a fire. There also needs to be a phone nearby in case of fire or some other type of emergency, to call 911.

You also need to give heed to home security. What happens if there is a burglary? The last thing in the world you would want would be for a loved one to be confronted by a dangerous intruder. Make sure there are deadbolts (though not requiring a key from the inside) on all of the doors, and reliable locks on the windows. You can also install motion detectors in the driveway to help deter burglars. This system will also make sure that the lights go on if you need to leave the house for any reason, especially in an emergency situation.

For maximum peace of mind, you may want to consider 24 hour monitoring. I'm referring to those "help, I've fallen and can't get up" devices we've all seen advertised on TV so much. These devices can usually be received for free if you qualify for Medicaid, and for a person needing assistance they can be a true lifesaver. For example, if a caregiver does not show up and the person cannot get out of bed they can press a button and get help immediately. It either triggers a pre-recorded message or opens up a speaker phone so they can instantly be connected to someone who can help them. These are known as emergency call buttons. I know of several clients who have horror stories of being left alone by previous agencies, with no way of being able to call for help. In one of these very unfortunate situations, these clever little devices could without question be lifesaving.

I might add that you should also have a neighbor or someone nearby who can go over and check on the person requiring care if there is some type of (non-emergency) situation, but you can't get over there quickly enough. Just be careful not to take advantage of this neighbor's generosity. As we mentioned earlier, be sure to reserve your calls to these people only for really serious situations. This person's number could also be on file with the automatic monitoring service so they can be notified if there is some sort of problem.

One last area of home safety we need to address is the "hidden" side of home health care. It is hidden because it is so shameful. What I'm talking about is abuse. Ironically, abuse is a major concern of people who fear going into a nursing home. How terrible it would be to successfully stay out of the nursing home, only to be abused in your own house! It is your responsibility to make sure it doesn't happen in your home, or to someone you love. If the person receiving care is managing their own caregivers and is mentally sharp, there may be nothing needed. That person in all likelihood can take care of him or herself.

However, it is quite a different story when the person being cared for is someone who is easily intimidated or unable to communicate any abuse that might be happening. In these cases, I would suggest that you take proactive measures. Let modern technology ease your burden. I know of a place locally named the Spy Shop that can keep an eye on your home surreptitiously for $1,000 (installed). A small price to pay, really, when you consider what you receive in return. The knowledge that any abuse will soon be discovered and immediately stopped.

Here's how it works. The cameras are set up in different parts of the house in such a way that nobody would have any way of knowing they are there. They are hooked up to a specially made Video Cassette Recorder for which you only have to change the tapes once per month. They can install the VCR in a closet or an attic so no one knows of the precaution being taken. This way if you suspect abuse or theft you can look back over the tape to verify your suspicions – and you now have proof to prosecute this person with so they can't victimize anyone else.

Of course, you only need to install cameras if you're beginning to get concerned that there might be a problem. It's the exact same reasoning that parents have for installing the now popular Nanny cam. They want to know that the loved one they are leaving in the care of a stranger is being treated properly and not being taken advantage of in any way. Remember the story I told you earlier about the gentleman who suspected that his mother's caregiver was stealing things from her house? Well, if he had had one of these cameras he would have had irrefutable proof to nail her. This would have saved him the cost of the unemployment he had to pay her...which was more than what he would have paid to buy the camera. A win-win situation for everyone, except the abuser.

Thankfully, the vast majority of caregivers are not abusive in any way. In fact, viewing the tapes could be an ideal way for you to see first hand what a great job they do, and how hard they work. You don't have to tell them that you saw their good work on tape, of course, but the next time you encounter this person it might be a nice gesture to let her know how much you appreciate all that she does for your loved one. Just exactly how you know she does such a good job will have to remain your own little secret.

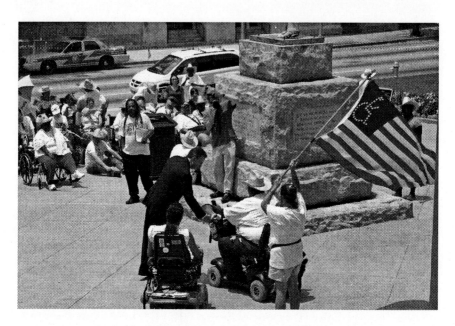

And a little more talk with politicians.

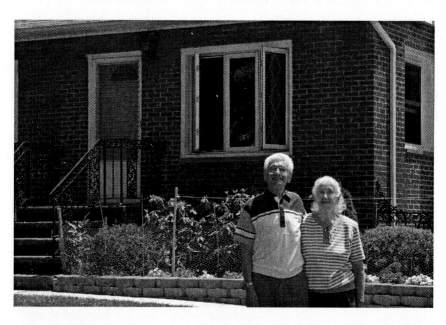

Ottaviano's enjoying a day with their grandson, I was taking the photo.

About the Author:

Dominic Ottaviano's extensive background in human resources and insurance play a vital role giving him the unique ability to combine his entrepreneurial success to home health care management. Dominic became friends with Zen Garcia in 1997 which allowed him to gather insight into the disability community to which he applied his business zest to improve care for persons with disabilities by allowing them to hire better caregivers and increase their quality of life. Dominic is a SCUBA Instructor introducing persons with disabilities to the wonderful world of undersea weightlessness, enjoys photography by capturing the beauty in our world, and is an accomplished pilot looking for the next adventure.

Printed in the United States
37012LVS00005B/295-312